INTERMITTENT FASTING FOR WOMEN OVER 50

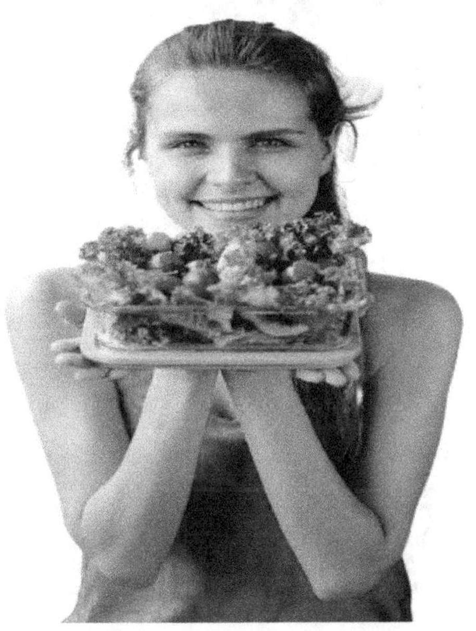

Dr. Mary Dixon

Copyright © 2023 by Dr. Mary Dixon

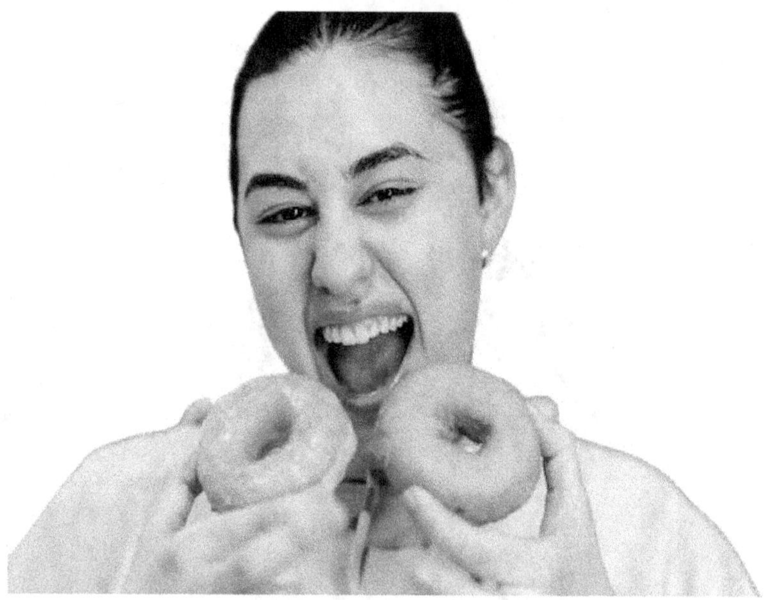

Table of Contents

INTRODUCTION

Meet Sarah. Sarah had always struggled with her weight and had tried countless diets and exercise routines over the years, but nothing seemed to work for her.

She was frustrated and discouraged, feeling like she was destined to be overweight and unhealthy for the rest of her life.

One day, a friend suggested she try intermittent fasting. Sarah was sceptical at first, but her friend explained that intermittent fasting had been shown to have a wide range of health benefits, including weight loss, improved blood sugar control, and reduced inflammation.

With nothing to lose, Sarah decided to give it a try. She started by fasting for 16 hours each day, only eating during an 8-hour window.

At first, it was challenging, and Sarah felt hungry and irritable during her fasting periods. But after a few days, her body adjusted, and she started to feel more energized and focused.

After a few weeks of intermittent fasting, Sarah started to notice a difference in her weight and overall health. She had lost a few pounds, and her clothes were fitting better. Her energy levels had improved, and she no longer felt sluggish and tired all the time.

Encouraged by her progress, Sarah decided to continue with intermittent fasting. She gradually increased the length of her fasting periods, eventually settling on a 20-hour fast each day.

She found that this routine worked well for her, and she was able to stick to it without feeling deprived or hungry.

Sarah's health kept getting better over time. She no longer struggled with high blood sugar, and her inflammation levels had gone down.

Her mood had improved, and she felt more confident and in control of her life.

Today, Sarah is a firm believer in the power of intermittent fasting. She has achieved good health, and she continues to maintain her fasting routine as part of her daily life.

She's proud of the progress she's made, and she hopes that her story will inspire others to try intermittent fasting and achieve their health goals.

Intermittent fasting has become a popular dietary trend in recent years, with many people incorporating it into their lifestyle as a way to improve their overall health and wellbeing.

The basic principle of intermittent fasting involves cycling between periods of eating and fasting, with the goal of providing a variety of benefits for the body and mind.

For women over 50, intermittent fasting can be particularly beneficial, as it can help to address some of the unique health challenges that may arise as they age.

As women approach menopause, they may experience a range of hormonal changes that can impact their metabolism and energy levels, making it more difficult to maintain a healthy weight and overall wellness.

Intermittent fasting offers a potential solution to these challenges, as it can help to boost metabolism, increase energy levels, and promote weight loss.

Additionally, research has shown that intermittent fasting can provide a range of other benefits for women over 50, including improved cognitive function, better sleep, and a lower risk of developing chronic illnesses including diabetes, heart disease, and some forms of cancer.

Of course, as with any dietary approach, it is important for women over 50 to approach intermittent fasting with caution and to consult with their healthcare provider before making any significant changes to their diet or lifestyle.

However, for those who are able to safely incorporate intermittent fasting into their routine, it can be a powerful tool for improving overall health and wellbeing in later life.

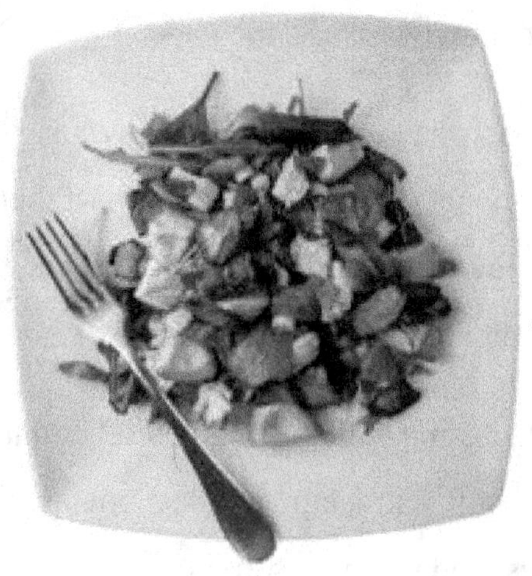

CHAPTER ONE

Intermittent Fasting for Women Over 50 Explained

Intermittent fasting (IF) has been gaining popularity in recent years as a way to improve overall health, lose weight, and even increase longevity.

However, many women over 50 may wonder if (IF) is a safe and effective diet strategy for their age group. In this book, we will explore the benefits and potential risks of IF for women over 50, as well as provide some tips for incorporating IF into your diet.

What is Intermittent Fasting?

Intermittent fasting is a dietary approach that involves cycling between periods of fasting and periods of eating.

Risks of Intermittent Fasting for Women Over 50

While there are many potential benefits of IF, there are also some potential risks, especially for women over 50.

Some of these risks include:

1. **Hormonal Imbalances:** Women over 50 may be more susceptible to hormonal imbalances due to the changes that occur during menopause. IF may exacerbate these imbalances and lead to irregular menstrual cycles or other hormonal issues.

2. **Nutrient Deficiencies:** IF may make it more difficult for women over 50 to get the nutrients they need, especially if they are not eating a balanced diet during their eating windows.

3. **Increased Risk of Osteoporosis:** Women over 50 are already at an increased risk of osteoporosis, and IF may exacerbate this risk by reducing bone density.

4. **Increased Risk of Gallstones:** Fasting can increase the risk of gallstones, especially in women over 50.

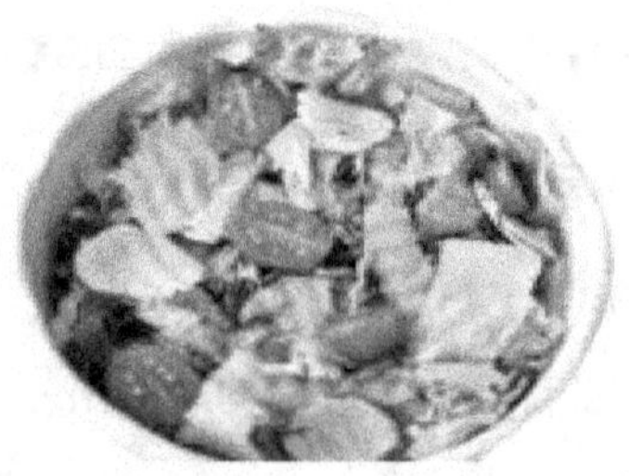

Guidelines for Including Intermittent Fasting in Your Diet

If you are interested in trying IF, here are some tips to help you get started:

1. **Start Slowly:** If you have never fasted before, start with a shorter fasting window and gradually increase it over time.

2. **Stay Hydrated:** Make sure to drink plenty of water and other non-caloric beverages during your fasting periods.

3. **Choose Nutrient-Dense Foods:** When you are eating, focus on nutrient-dense foods like fruits, vegetables, whole grains, and lean protein sources.

4. **Consider a Modified Approach:** Instead of a strict fasting schedule, you may want to consider a modified approach that involves reducing your calorie intake during certain times of the day or week.

5. **Consult with Your Doctor:** Before starting any new diet or exercise program, it is important to consult with your doctor, especially if you have any underlying health conditions.

6. **Listen to Your Body:** Pay attention to how your body responds to IF and adjust your approach as needed. If you feel dizzy, weak, or overly hungry, it may be a sign that IF is not the right approach for you.

7. **Combine with Exercise:** Combining IF with exercise can help to boost weight loss and improve overall health. However, it is important to make sure you are getting enough nutrients and calories to support your exercise routine.

Intermittent fasting can be a safe and effective diet strategy for women over 50, but it is important to approach it with caution and make sure you are getting the nutrients and calories you need to support your health.

As with any diet or exercise program, it is important to consult with your doctor before getting started.

By following these tips and listening to your body, you can incorporate IF into your diet and reap the potential benefits it has to offer.

Types of Intermittent Fasting for Women Over 50

There are several different methods of IF, including:

1. **16/8 Method:** The 16/8 Method calls for a 16-hour period of fasting and an 8-hour interval for eating.

2. **5:2 Method:** Using the 5:2 method, you eat normally for 5 days and then limit your caloric intake to 500–600 for 2 separate, non-consecutive days.

3. **Alternate Day Fasting:** This involves eating normally on non-fasting days while fasting every other day.

4. **Eat-Stop-Eat Method:** This entails going without food once or twice a week for 24 hours.

5. **The Warrior Diet:** The Warrior Diet involves eating one large meal at night and fasting during the day.

Some people on this diet also eat a small amount of raw fruits and vegetables during the day.

It is important for women over 50 to consult with their healthcare provider before starting any new dietary strategy, including intermittent fasting.

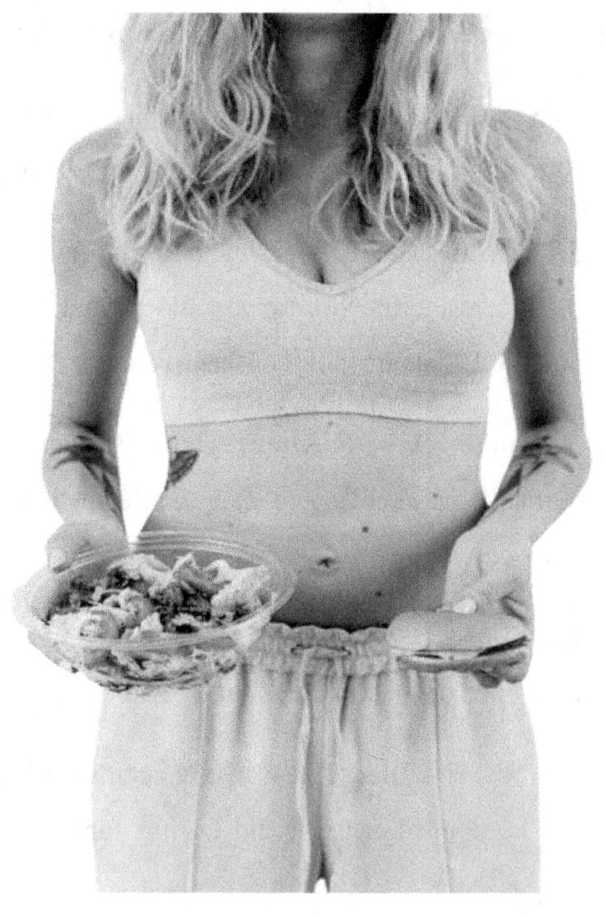

CHAPTER TWO

Intermittent Fasting for Women Over 50 Diet and Benefits

Intermittent fasting has become a popular way of eating in recent years, with many people turning to this lifestyle for weight loss and other health benefits.

Alternating between eating and fasting is known as intermittent fasting. While the practice has been around for centuries, it has gained more popularity in recent years with the emergence of various scientific studies backing up its numerous benefits.

Intermittent fasting is a lifestyle that has been found to be beneficial for women over 50. This is because as women age, their metabolism slows down, making it more difficult to maintain a healthy weight.

Intermittent fasting is a great way for women over 50 to boost their metabolism, lose weight, and improve their overall health.

Intermittent fasting can be done in a variety of ways. One of the most popular methods is the 16/8 method. In this approach, a 16-hour fast is followed by an 8-hour interval for eating. For example, you might skip breakfast and eat your first meal at noon and then finish eating by 8 p.m.

Another popular method is the 5:2 diet, where you eat normally for five days of the week and then restrict calories to 500-600 for the remaining two days.

So, what are the benefits of intermittent fasting for women over 50?

Weight Loss

Weight loss is one of the main advantages of intermittent fasting. As we age, it becomes increasingly difficult to lose weight and keep it off. Intermittent fasting has been shown to be effective for weight loss because it reduces the number of calories you consume. By fasting for a certain number of hours each day or week, you can create a calorie deficit, which will result in weight loss.

Reduced Inflammation

Intermittent fasting has also been found to reduce inflammation in the body. Numerous health issues, including as heart disease, cancer, and Alzheimer's disease, are associated with inflammation. By reducing inflammation, intermittent fasting may help prevent these diseases and improve overall health.

Improved Brain Function

Intermittent fasting has been found to improve brain function and protect against age-related cognitive decline. Studies have shown that intermittent fasting can increase the production of brain-derived neurotrophic factor (BDNF), which is a protein that is essential for brain health.

Reduced Risk of Type 2 Diabetes

Intermittent fasting has been shown to improve insulin sensitivity, which can help reduce the risk of type 2 diabetes. Insulin sensitivity is the ability of your body to respond to insulin, which is essential for regulating blood sugar levels.

By improving insulin sensitivity, intermittent fasting can help prevent type 2 diabetes.

Improved Heart Health

Intermittent fasting has been found to improve heart health by reducing blood pressure, triglycerides, and LDL cholesterol levels. High blood pressure, high triglycerides, and high LDL cholesterol are all risk factors for heart disease. By reducing these risk factors, intermittent fasting can help improve heart health and reduce the risk of heart disease.

Improved Immune System Function

Intermittent fasting has also been found to improve immune system function. By reducing inflammation and improving overall health, intermittent fasting can help boost the immune system, making it more effective at fighting off infections and diseases.

Longevity

Finally, intermittent fasting has been found to increase lifespan in animals. While more research is needed in humans, the potential for increased lifespan is an exciting benefit of intermittent fasting.

While there are many benefits to intermittent fasting, it is important to note that it may not be suitable for everyone. Intermittent fasting should not be done by pregnant or nursing women. Women with a history of eating disorders should also be cautious and talk to their doctor before trying intermittent fasting.

In conclusion, intermittent fasting is a great way for women over 50 to improve their health and well-being. It can aid in weight loss, reduce inflammation, improve brain function, reduce the risk of type 2 diabetes and heart disease, improve immune system function, and potentially increase lifespan.

If you are considering intermittent fasting, it is important to start slowly and consult with your doctor or a registered dietitian to ensure that it is appropriate for you.

It is also important to ensure that you are consuming enough calories and nutrients during your eating periods to maintain good health.

In addition to intermittent fasting, it is important for women over 50 to maintain a healthy diet, exercise regularly, get enough sleep, and manage stress.

These lifestyle factors, in addition to intermittent fasting, can help improve overall health and well-being and reduce the risk of chronic diseases.

Overall, intermittent fasting is a promising lifestyle change for women over 50. With its numerous health benefits, it can help promote a healthier and more fulfilling life.

How to Follow an Intermittent Fasting for Women Over 50 Diet

A nutritional strategy known as intermittent fasting involves alternating between periods of fasting and eating.

It has gained popularity over the years due to its potential health benefits, including weight loss, improved metabolism, and reduced inflammation.

However, women over 50 may have unique nutritional needs that need to be considered when following an intermittent fasting diet.

In this book, we will discuss how to follow an intermittent fasting diet for women over 50.

Consult with a healthcare professional:

Before starting any new diet or exercise regimen, it is important to consult with a healthcare professional. Women over 50 may have underlying health conditions that need to be considered before starting an intermittent fasting diet. It is also important to discuss any medications that you are taking, as some medications may need to be adjusted with changes in diet and lifestyle.

Choose the right fasting schedule:

There are different types of intermittent fasting schedules, including the 16/8 method, the 5:2 diet, and alternate-day fasting. For women over 50, it may be beneficial to start with a less restrictive schedule, such as the 16/8 method. This entails a 16-hour period of fasting and an 8-hour window for eating. It is important to listen to your body and adjust the fasting schedule as needed.

Focus on nutrient-dense foods:

When following an intermittent fasting diet, it is important to choose nutrient-dense foods that provide essential vitamins and minerals. This can include lean protein, whole grains, fruits, vegetables, and healthy fats. Women over 50 may also benefit from increasing their intake of calcium and vitamin D to support bone health.

Stay hydrated:

During fasting periods, it is important to stay hydrated by drinking plenty of water, herbal tea, and other non-caloric beverages. Women over 50 may also benefit from increasing their intake of electrolytes, such as sodium, potassium, and magnesium, to support overall health.

Avoid processed foods and added sugars:

To maximize the potential health benefits of intermittent fasting, it is important to avoid processed foods and added sugars. These can contribute to inflammation, insulin resistance, and other health issues. Instead, focus on whole, unprocessed foods that provide essential nutrients and support overall health.

Consider supplements:

Women over 50 may benefit from taking supplements to support their nutritional needs during intermittent fasting. This can include a high-quality multivitamin, omega-3 fatty acids, and probiotics to support gut health.

Listen to your body:

It is important to listen to your body when following an intermittent fasting diet. Women over 50 may have unique nutritional needs that need to be considered, and it is important to adjust the fasting schedule and food choices as needed. If you experience any negative side effects, such as fatigue, dizziness, or headaches, it may be necessary to modify your approach or consult with a healthcare professional.Intermittent fasting can be a safe and effective dietary approach for women over 50. By choosing the right fasting schedule, focusing on nutrient-dense foods, staying hydrated, avoiding processed foods and added sugars, considering supplements, and listening to your body, you can maximize the potential health benefits of intermittent fasting and support your overall health and well-being.

As usual, before adopting any significant dietary or lifestyle changes, you should speak with a healthcare provider.

7 Day Intermittent Fasting for Women Over 50

Day 1

12 pm:

Greek Salad with Grilled Chicken

Combine chopped romaine lettuce, cherry tomatoes, sliced cucumbers, red onion, kalamata olives, and feta cheese. Top with grilled chicken and a drizzle of olive oil and red wine vinegar.

4 pm:

Raw Vegetables with Hummus

Slice up raw vegetables like carrots, celery, and bell peppers and serve with hummus for dipping.

7 pm:

Grilled Salmon with Roasted Vegetables

Season salmon fillets with salt, pepper, and garlic powder and grill until cooked through. Serve with roasted vegetables like Brussels sprouts, cauliflower, and sweet potatoes.

Day 2

12 pm:

Avocado and Egg Toast

Toast a slice of whole-grain bread and top with mashed avocado, a poached egg, and a sprinkle of Everything Bagel seasoning.

4 pm:

Apple Slices with Almond Butter

Slice up an apple and serve with almond butter for dipping.

7 pm:

Turkey Chili –

Brown ground turkey in a large pot and add diced onion, diced bell pepper, minced garlic, and canned tomatoes. Season with chili powder, cumin, and paprika. Simmer until vegetables are tender and chili is heated through.

Day 3

12 pm:

Spinach and Feta Omelette

Whisk together eggs, chopped spinach, crumbled feta cheese, and a dash of milk. Cook in a non-stick pan until set.

4 pm:

Greek Yogurt with Berries

Mix Greek yogurt with fresh berries and a drizzle of honey.

7 pm:

Grilled Chicken Caesar Salad

Grill chicken and chop into bite-sized pieces. Combine with chopped romaine lettuce, croutons, and Caesar dressing.

Day 4

12 pm:

Smoked Salmon and Cream Cheese Bagel

Toast a whole-grain bagel and spread with cream cheese. Top with smoked salmon, sliced cucumber, and red onion.

4 pm:

Nuts and Dried Fruit

Mix together a variety of nuts and dried fruit like almonds, cashews, and raisins.

7 pm:

Grilled Shrimp Skewers with Zucchini Noodles

Skewer peeled and deveined shrimp and grill until cooked through. Serve with spiralized zucchini noodles and a drizzle of olive oil and lemon juice.

Day 5

12 pm:

Southwest Salad with Chicken

Combine chopped romaine lettuce, canned black beans, corn, diced tomatoes, and shredded chicken. Top with a dollop of Greek yogurt and a sprinkle of chili powder.

4 pm:

Cheese and Crackers

Serve a variety of cheese with whole-grain crackers.

7 pm:

Beef Stir-Fry with Vegetables

Slice beef thinly and stir-fry with vegetables like bell peppers, broccoli, and carrots. Serve with brown rice.

Day 6

12 pm:

Green Smoothie Bowl

Blend together spinach, frozen mixed berries, banana, Greek yogurt, and almond milk. Pour into a bowl and top with sliced fruit, granola, and a drizzle of honey.

4 pm:

Hard-Boiled Eggs with Salt and Pepper

Boil eggs and serve with a sprinkle of salt and pepper.

7 pm:

Baked Salmon with Asparagus

Place salmon fillets and asparagus spears on a baking sheet and drizzle with olive oil and lemon juice. Cook in the oven until fully done.

Day 7

12 pm:

Banana and Peanut Butter Oatmeal

Cook oats according to package instructions and top with sliced banana and a spoonful of peanut butter.

4 pm:

Vegetable Soup

Make a large pot of vegetable soup with vegetables like carrots, celery, onion, and zucchini. Serve with whole-grain crackers.

7 pm:

Turkey Burger with Sweet Potato Fries

Mix ground turkey with minced onion, garlic, and Worcestershire sauce. Form into patties and grill. Serve with sweet potato fries baked in the oven.

Additional Tips:

1. To stay hydrated during fasting, drink a lot of water.

2. During your eating window, focus on nutrient-dense whole foods like fruits, vegetables, lean proteins, and healthy fats.

3. Limit processed foods, sugary drinks, and alcohol.

4. If you have any health concerns or medical conditions, consult with a healthcare professional before starting an intermittent fasting protocol.

I hope this meal plan and tips are helpful in getting started with an intermittent fasting protocol.

It's important to listen to your body and adjust the plan as needed to fit your individual needs and preferences.

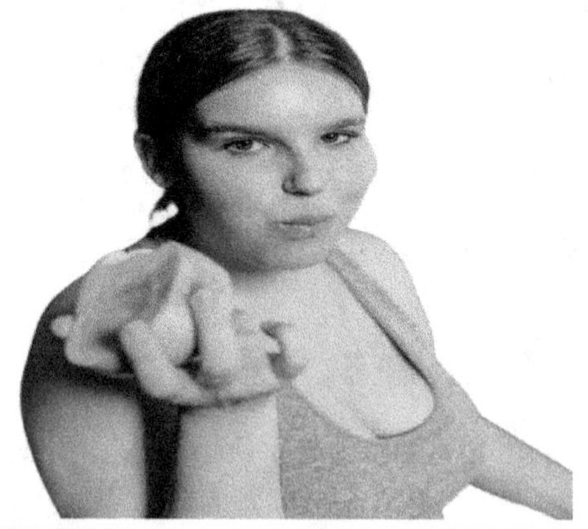

CHAPTER THREE

Intermittent Fasting for Women Over 50 Recipes

Breakfast

1. Avocado and Egg Toast

This recipe is packed with healthy fats and protein to keep you full throughout your fasting period.

Ingredients:

- 1 slice whole wheat bread

- 1/2 avocado

- 1 egg

- Salt and pepper to taste

Instructions:

1. Toasted bread should be as crisp as you like.

2. Spread the avocado on the toast after mashing it.

3. Place the egg on top of the avocado after frying it to the desired doneness.

4. Serve right away after adding salt and pepper on the top.

Cooking Time: 10 minutes

2. Greek Yogurt Parfait

This recipe is a quick and easy way to get a dose of protein and probiotics.

Ingredients:

- 1 cup Greek yogurt

- 1/2 cup mixed berries

- 1/4 cup granola

Instructions:

1. Layer the yogurt, berries, and granola in a jar or bowl.

2. Repeat until you reach the top.

3. Serve immediately.

Cooking Time: 5 minutes

3. Sweet Potato Hash with Eggs

This recipe is a hearty and satisfying breakfast that is perfect for the colder months.

Ingredients:

- 1 sweet potato

- 1/2 onion

- 2 eggs

- Salt and pepper to taste

Instructions:

1. Sweet potato and onion should be peeled and diced.

2. Heat a non-stick skillet over medium heat.

3. Add the sweet potato and onion and cook until softened, stirring occasionally.

4. Crack the eggs over the top of the hash and cover the skillet.

5. Cook until the eggs reach the desired doneness.

6. Season with salt and pepper and serve.

Cooking Time: 20 minutes

4. Chia Seed Pudding

This recipe is a great way to get a dose of fibre and omega-3s in the morning.

Ingredients:

- 1/2 cup chia seeds

- 2 cups unsweetened almond milk

- 1/4 cup honey

- 1 tsp vanilla extract

Instructions:

1. Chia seeds, almond milk, honey, and vanilla extract should all be combined in a bowl.

2. Let the mixture sit for at least 30 minutes, or until it thickens to a pudding-like consistency.

3. Serve chilled.

Cooking Time: 30 minutes

5. Scrambled Eggs with Spinach

This recipe is a great way to get a dose of leafy greens in the morning.

Ingredients:

- 2 eggs

- 1 cup baby spinach

- Salt and pepper to taste

Instructions:

1. Add salt and pepper to the beaten eggs before beating them in a bowl.

2. A non-stick skillet should be heated to medium.

3. Baby spinach should be added and cooked until wilted.

4. Scramble the eggs by pouring them over the spinach.

5. Serve after adding more salt and pepper, if desired.

Cooking Time: 10 minutes

6. Green Smoothie

This recipe is a great way to get a dose of fruits and veggies in the morning.

Ingredients:

- 1 banana

- 1 cup spinach

- 1/2 cup frozen pineapple

- 1/2 cup unsweetened almond milk

Instructions:

1. Combine all ingredients in a blender.

2. Blend until smooth.

3. Serve immediately.

Cooking Time: 5 minutes

7. Cottage Cheese with Fruit

This recipe is a quick and easy way to get a dose of protein and fruit in the morning.

Ingredients:

- 1/2 cup cottage cheese

- 1/2 cup mixed berries

Instructions:

1. Spoon the cottage cheese into a bowl.

2. Top with mixed berries.

3. Serve immediately.

Cooking Time: 5 minutes

8. Smoked Salmon and Cream Cheese on Whole Wheat Toast

This recipe is a delicious way to get a dose of omega-3s and protein in the morning.

Ingredients:

- 1 slice whole wheat bread

- 2 oz smoked salmon

- 2 tbsp cream cheese

Instructions:

1. Toasted bread should be as crisp as you like.

2. Spread the cream cheese onto the toast.

3. Place the smoked salmon on top of the cream cheese.

4. Serve immediately.

Cooking Time: 5 minutes

9. Quinoa Breakfast Bowl

This recipe is a filling and nutritious way to start your day.

Ingredients:

- 1/2 cup cooked quinoa

- 1/4 cup sliced almonds

- 1/4 cup dried cranberries

- 1/4 cup unsweetened almond milk

- 1 tsp honey

Instructions:

1. Combine the quinoa, almonds, and dried cranberries in a bowl.

2. Drizzle the almond milk and honey over the top.

3. Stir to combine.

4. Serve chilled.

Cooking Time: 15 minutes

10. Omelette with Vegetables

This recipe is a great way to get a dose of protein and vegetables in the morning.

Ingredients:

- 2 eggs

- 1/2 bell pepper, diced

- 1/4 onion, diced

- Salt and pepper to taste

Instructions:

1. Add salt and pepper to the beaten eggs before beating them in a bowl.

2. A non-stick skillet should be heated to medium.

3. Bell pepper and onion should be added and cooked until tender.

4. Pour the eggs over the vegetables and cook until set.

5. Fold the omelette in half and serve.

Cooking Time: 15 minutes

I hope you enjoy these intermittent fasting breakfast recipes! Remember to adjust portion sizes and ingredients to fit your specific dietary needs.

CHAPTER FOUR

Lunch

1. Grilled Chicken and Vegetable Salad

This salad is perfect for a low-carb lunch option. The chicken and vegetables are grilled for a smoky flavour and paired with a tangy dressing.

Ingredients:

- 1 boneless chicken breast

- 1 zucchini, sliced

- 1 yellow squash, sliced

- 1/2 red onion, sliced

- 2 cups mixed greens

- 2 tablespoons olive oil

- 1 tablespoon balsamic vinegar

- Salt and pepper to taste

Instructions:

1. Preheat the grill to medium-high heat.

2. Season the chicken breast with salt and pepper. Grill for 6-8 minutes on each side, until fully cooked.

3. In a separate bowl, toss the sliced zucchini, yellow squash, and red onion with 1 tablespoon of olive oil. Grill each side for three to four minutes.

4. In a large bowl, mix the mixed greens with the remaining tablespoon of olive oil and balsamic vinegar.

5. Add the grilled vegetables and sliced chicken on top of the salad. Serve and enjoy.

Cooking Time: 20-25 minutes

2. Chickpea Salad with Feta and Cucumber

This refreshing salad is packed with protein and fibre from the chickpeas, and the feta cheese adds a creamy texture.

Ingredients:

- 1 can chickpeas, drained and rinsed
- 1/2 cucumber, diced
- 1/2 red onion, diced
- 1/4 cup crumbled feta cheese
- 2 tablespoons olive oil
- 1 tablespoon red wine vinegar
- Salt and pepper to taste

Instructions:

1. In a large bowl, mix the chickpeas, cucumber, red onion, and feta cheese.

2. Whisk the olive oil, red wine vinegar, salt, and pepper in a separate basin.

3. After adding the dressing, toss the salad to incorporate.

4. Serve and enjoy.

Cooking Time: 10 minutes

3. Turkey and Avocado Lettuce Wraps

These lettuce wraps are a healthy, low-carb alternative to traditional wraps or sandwiches.

Ingredients:

- 1 pound ground turkey

- 1 avocado, mashed

- 1/2 red onion, diced

- 1/2 red bell pepper, diced

- 1 tablespoon olive oil

- Salt and pepper to taste

- Butter lettuce leaves

Instructions:

1. Olive oil should be heated to a medium-high temperature in a big skillet.

2. Add the salt, pepper, and ground turkey to the mixture. Cook for 8 to 10 minutes or until thoroughly done.

3. Remove the skillet from heat and mix in the mashed avocado.

4. Spoon the turkey and avocado mixture onto the butter lettuce leaves.

5. Roll up the leaves and secure with toothpicks, if desired. Serve and enjoy.

Cooking Time: 15-20 minutes

4. Shrimp and Broccoli Stir-Fry

This stir-fry is a quick and easy lunch option that is packed with protein and fibre from the shrimp and broccoli.

Ingredients:

- 1 pound shrimp, peeled and deveined

- 2 cups broccoli florets

- 1 red bell pepper, sliced

- 1/2 red onion, sliced

- 2 cloves garlic, minced

- 2 tablespoons soy sauce

- 1 tablespoon honey

- 1 tablespoon corn-starch

- 1 tablespoon sesame oil

- Salt and pepper to taste

Instructions:

1. In a small bowl, whisk together the soy sauce, honey, corn-starch, and 1 tablespoon of sesame oil. Set aside.

2. In a large skillet or wok, heat the remaining tablespoon of sesame oil over high heat.

3. Add the shrimp and cook for 2-3 minutes on each side, until pink and fully cooked. Take out of the skillet, then set it aside.

4. Add the broccoli, red bell pepper, red onion, and garlic to the skillet. Vegetables should be stir-fried for 3–4 minutes or until they are crisp-tender.

5. Add the shrimp back to the skillet, along with the soy sauce mixture. For a further minute, stir-fry, or until the sauce thickens.

6. Serve and enjoy.

Cooking Time: 15-20 minutes

5. Cauliflower Fried Rice with Tofu

This cauliflower fried rice is a healthy and low-carb alternative to traditional fried rice. The tofu adds protein and texture to the dish.

Ingredients:

- 1 head cauliflower, grated or pulsed in a food processor

- 1 block tofu, drained and pressed

- 2 cloves garlic, minced

- 1/2 onion, diced

- 1 cup frozen peas and carrots

- 2 tablespoons soy sauce

- 1 tablespoon sesame oil

- Salt and pepper to taste

Instructions:

1. Heat the sesame oil over medium-high heat in a big skillet or wok.

2. Crumble the tofu into the skillet and cook for 5-7 minutes, until lightly browned.

3. Add the garlic and onion to the skillet and cook for another 2-3 minutes, until the onion is translucent.

4. Stir-fry the frozen peas and carrots for two to three minutes in the skillet.

5. Add the grated cauliflower to the skillet and stir-fry for another 2-3 minutes, until the cauliflower is tender.

6. Add the soy sauce and salt and pepper to taste. Stir
    to combine.

7. Serve and enjoy.

Cooking Time: 20-25 minutes

6. Spinach and Feta Stuffed Chicken Breast

This stuffed chicken breast is a delicious and healthy lunch
option that is packed with flavour.

Ingredients:

- 2 boneless chicken breasts

- 2 cups spinach leaves, chopped

- 1/4 cup crumbled feta cheese

- 2 cloves garlic, minced

- 2 tablespoons olive oil

- Salt and pepper to taste

Instructions:

1. Preheat the oven to 375°F (190°C).

2. Cut a pocket into each chicken breast at its thickest point with a sharp knife.

3. Combine the chopped spinach, feta cheese, garlic, 1 tablespoon of olive oil, salt, and pepper in a small bowl.

4. Place a small amount of spinach and feta in each chicken breast pocket.

5. Over medium-high heat, warm the last tablespoon of olive oil in a big skillet.

6. For two to three minutes on each side, brown the stuffed chicken breasts in the skillet.

7. Place the chicken breasts in a baking dish and cook them in the preheated oven for 20 to 25 minutes, depending on how done you like your chicken.

8. Serve and enjoy.

Cooking Time: 30-35 minutes

7. Tuna Salad Lettuce Wraps

These lettuce wraps are a low-carb and protein-packed lunch option that is perfect for a hot summer day.

Ingredients:

- 2 cans tuna, drained

- 1/4 cup diced celery

- 1/4 cup diced red onion

- 2 tablespoons mayonnaise

- 1 tablespoon lemon juice

- Salt and pepper to taste

- Butter lettuce leaves

Instructions:

1. In a large bowl, mix together the tuna, celery, red onion, mayonnaise, lemon juice, salt, and pepper.

2. Spoon the tuna salad mixture onto butter lettuce leaves.

3. Roll up the lettuce leaves and secure with toothpicks,
   if desired.

4. Serve and enjoy.

Cooking Time: 10-15 minutes

8. Turkey and Avocado Lettuce Wraps

These lettuce wraps are a healthy and delicious lunch option
that is packed with protein and healthy fats.

Ingredients:

- 1 pound ground turkey

- 1/2 onion, diced

- 1 avocado, diced

- 2 tablespoons olive oil

- Salt and pepper to taste

- Butter lettuce leaves

Instructions:

1. Olive oil should be heated to a medium-high temperature in a big skillet.

2. Add the diced onion to the skillet and cook for 2-3 minutes, until the onion is translucent.

3. Add the ground turkey to the skillet and cook for 5-7 minutes, until browned and fully cooked.

4. Add the diced avocado to the skillet and stir to combine.

5. Spoon the turkey and avocado mixture onto butter lettuce leaves.

6. Roll up the lettuce leaves and secure with toothpicks, if desired.

7. Serve and enjoy.

Cooking Time: 20-25 minutes

9. Grilled Chicken and Vegetable Kabobs

These grilled chicken and vegetable kabobs are a delicious and healthy lunch option that is perfect for summertime.

Ingredients:

- 2 boneless chicken breasts, divided into morsels

- 1 red onion, diced into small pieces.

- 1 red bell pepper, diced into small pieces.

- 1 zucchini, cut into bite-sized pieces

- 1/4 cup olive oil

- 2 tablespoons balsamic vinegar

- 1 tablespoon Dijon mustard

- Salt and pepper to taste

- Wooden or metal skewers

Instructions:

1. Soak wooden skewers in water for 30 minutes before grilling, if using.

2. Mix the olive oil, balsamic vinegar, Dijon mustard, salt, and pepper in a small bowl.

3. Chicken and vegetables are skewered together.

4. Apply the olive oil mixture to the skewers.

5. Grill the skewers over medium-high heat for 8-10 minutes, turning occasionally, until the chicken is fully cooked.

6. Serve and enjoy.

Cooking Time: 20-25 minutes

10. Salmon and Quinoa Salad

This salmon and quinoa salad is a healthy and satisfying lunch option that is packed with protein and omega-3 fatty acids.

Ingredients:

- 1 pound salmon fillet

- 1 cup cooked quinoa

- 2 cups mixed greens

- 1/2 red onion, thinly sliced

- 1/2 cucumber, diced

- 1/4 cup olive oil

- 2 tablespoons lemon juice

- Salt and pepper to taste

Instructions:

1. Preheat the oven to 375°F (190°C).

2. On a baking sheet covered with parchment paper, put the salmon fillet.

3. Salt and pepper the fish after drizzling it with olive oil.

4. Bake the salmon in the preheated oven for 12-15 minutes, until fully cooked.

5. In a large bowl, mix together the cooked quinoa, mixed greens, red onion, cucumber, olive oil, lemon juice, salt, and pepper.

6. The cooked salmon should be flaked and added to the salad.

7. Toss to combine.

8. Serve and enjoy.

Cooking Time: 25-30 minutes

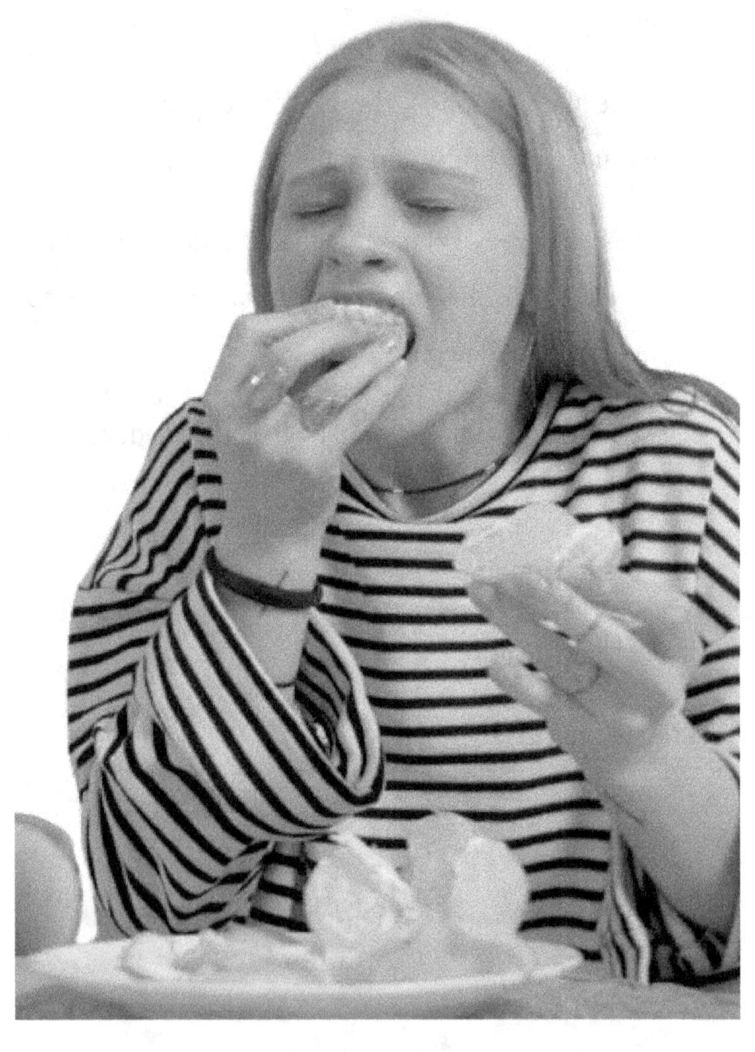

CHAPTER FIVE

Dinner

1. Lemon Garlic Shrimp and Asparagus

This dish is light, flavourful, and perfect for a summer evening. The shrimp and asparagus are both low in calories and high in protein, making it an ideal meal for intermittent fasting.

Ingredients:

- 1-pound large shrimp, peeled and deveined

- 1 bunch of trimmed and divided into 2-inch pieces asparagus

- 2 cloves garlic, minced

- 2 tablespoons olive oil

- 1 lemon, juiced and zested

- Salt and pepper to taste

Instructions:

1. Preheat the oven to 400°F (205°C).

2. In a bowl, combine the shrimp, asparagus, garlic, olive oil, lemon juice, lemon zest, salt, and pepper. Toss to combine.

3. On a baking sheet, distribute the mixture in a single layer.

4. Roast for 12-15 minutes, until the shrimp are pink and the asparagus is tender.

Cooking Time: 15 minutes

2. Grilled Chicken with Roasted Vegetables

This grilled chicken with roasted vegetables is a delicious and satisfying meal that is low in carbs and high in protein. The flavour combination is sure to satisfy.

Ingredients:

- 4 boneless, skinless chicken breasts

- 1 large zucchini, sliced

- 1 red pepper, sliced

- 1 yellow pepper, sliced

- 1 onion, sliced

- 2 tablespoons olive oil

- 1 tablespoon dried oregano

- Salt and pepper to taste

Instructions:

1. Preheat the grill to medium-high heat.

2. In a large bowl, combine the chicken, zucchini, red pepper, yellow pepper, onion, olive oil, oregano, salt, and pepper. Toss to combine.

3. The chicken should be cooked through after grilling for 6 to 8 minutes on each side.

4. Roast the vegetables in a separate pan in the oven at 400°F (205°C) for 20-25 minutes, or until tender.

Cooking Time: 30 minutes

3. Baked Salmon with Broccoli and Cauliflower Rice

Salmon is a great source of protein and healthy fats, making it an ideal meal for intermittent fasting. Paired with broccoli and cauliflower rice, this dish is both healthy and delicious.

Ingredients:

- 4 salmon fillets

- 2 cups broccoli florets

- 2 cups cauliflower rice

- 2 tablespoons olive oil

- 1 tablespoon garlic powder

- Salt and pepper to taste

Instructions:

1. Preheat the oven to 400°F (205°C).

2. In a large bowl, combine the salmon, broccoli, cauliflower rice, olive oil, garlic powder, salt, and pepper. Toss to combine.

3. On a baking sheet, distribute the mixture in a single
    layer.

4. Bake for 15-20 minutes, or until the veggies are soft
    and the salmon is fully cooked.

Cooking Time: 20 minutes

4. Stuffed Bell Peppers

Stuffed bell peppers are a classic dish that is both healthy
and filling. This version is made with ground turkey, quinoa,
and lots of flavourful spices.

Ingredients:

- 4 bell peppers, halved and seeded

- 1 pound ground turkey

- 1 cup cooked quinoa

- 1 onion, diced

- 2 cloves garlic

- 1 teaspoon cumin

- 1 teaspoon chili powder

- 1/2 teaspoon paprika

- Salt and pepper to taste

Instructions:

1. Preheat the oven to 375°F (190°C).

2. Cook the ground turkey in a large skillet over medium-high heat.

3. Cook the onion and garlic in the skillet until they are tender.

4. Stir in the cooked quinoa, cumin, chili powder, paprika, salt, and pepper.

5. Arrange the bell pepper halves on a baking sheet and fill each half with the turkey mixture.

6. Bake the peppers for 25 to 30 minutes, or until they are soft and the filling is thoroughly cooked.

Cooking Time: 35 minutes

5. Spicy Tomato Soup with Croutons of Grilled Cheese

This tomato soup is kicked up a notch with some spice, and the grilled cheese croutons add a satisfying crunch.

Ingredients:

- 2 tablespoons olive oil

- 1 onion, diced

- 2 cloves garlic, minced

- 1 teaspoon red pepper flakes

- 1 can (28 ounces) diced tomatoes

- 1 cup chicken broth

- 1 teaspoon dried basil

- Salt and pepper to taste

- 4 slices whole grain bread

- 4 slices cheddar cheese

Instructions:

1. Olive oil should be heated in a sizable pot over a medium-high heat.

2. The onion and garlic should be added to the stew and cooked until tender.

3. Add the basil, red pepper flakes, diced tomatoes, chicken broth, salt, and pepper after stirring.

4. The mixture should be heated until it boils, then it should be simmered for 15 to 20 minutes.

5. Pre-heat the oven to 400°F (205°C) in the interim.

6. Place the bread on a baking pan after cutting it into small cubes.

7. Add a slice of cheddar cheese to the top of each bread cube.

8. Bake for 10 to 12 minutes, or until bubbling and melted cheese.

9. With the grilled cheese croutons on top, serve the soup hot.

Cooking Time: 30 minutes

6. Zucchini Noodle Stir Fry

Zucchini noodles make a great low-carb alternative to traditional noodles. This stir fry is loaded with veggies and protein, making it a well-rounded meal.

Ingredients:

- 4 zucchinis, spiralized

- 1 pound chicken breast, sliced

- 1 red bell pepper, sliced

- 1 yellow bell pepper, sliced

- 1 onion, sliced

- 2 cloves garlic, minced

- 2 tablespoons coconut oil

- 1 tablespoon soy sauce

- 1 tablespoon sesame oil

- Salt and pepper to taste

Instructions:

1. In a large skillet, heat the coconut oil over medium-high heat.

2. The chicken should be added to the skillet and cooked until browned all over.

3. Add the bell peppers, onion, and garlic to the skillet and cook until the veggies are softened.

4. Stir in the zucchini noodles, soy sauce, sesame oil, salt, and pepper.

5. Cook for an additional 5-7 minutes, or until the zucchini noodles are tender.

Cooking Time: 25 minutes

7. Turkey Meatballs with Marinara Sauce

These turkey meatballs are loaded with flavour and are a great source of protein. Paired with a simple marinara sauce, they make a delicious and satisfying meal.

Ingredients:

- 1 pound ground turkey

- 1/2 cup breadcrumbs

- 1/4 cup grated Parmesan cheese

- 1 egg

- 1/4 cup fresh parsley, chopped

- Salt and pepper to taste

- 1 jar (24 ounces) marinara sauce

Instructions:

1. Preheat the oven to 375°F (190°C).

2. Combine the ground turkey, breadcrumbs, Parmesan cheese, egg, parsley, salt, and pepper in a sizable mixing basin.

3. All of the ingredients should be thoroughly mixed.

4. Make little balls out of the mixture that are 1 inch in diameter or smaller.

5. On a baking sheet covered with parchment paper, arrange the meatballs.

6. Bake the meatballs for 20 to 25 minutes, or until done.

7. While the meatballs are cooking, heat the marinara sauce in a small saucepan over low heat.

8. Once the meatballs are cooked, add them to the marinara sauce and stir until they are fully coated.

9. Serve hot with a side of steamed vegetables or a salad.

Cooking Time: 30 minutes

8. Salmon and Asparagus Bake

This simple and healthy recipe features salmon fillets and asparagus baked together in a flavourful lemon and herb sauce.

Ingredients:

- 4 salmon fillets

- 1 bunch asparagus, trimmed

- 1 lemon, sliced

- 2 cloves garlic, minced

- 2 tablespoons olive oil

- 1 tablespoon dried basil

- Salt and pepper to taste

Instructions:

1. Preheat the oven to 375°F (190°C).

2. In a small mixing bowl, whisk together the olive oil, garlic, basil, salt, and pepper.

3. On a baking sheet, arrange the salmon fillets and asparagus.

4. Drizzle the olive oil mixture over the top of the salmon and asparagus.

5. Place a few slices of lemon on top of each salmon fillet.

6. Bake the salmon and asparagus for 15-20 minutes, or until they are both cooked through.

Cooking Time: 25 minutes

9. Stuffed Acorn Squash

This cosy and comforting dish features acorn squash stuffed with a flavourful mixture of ground beef, quinoa, and spices.

Ingredients:

- 2 acorn squash, halved and seeded

- 1 pound ground beef

- 1 cup cooked quinoa

- 1 onion, diced

- 2 cloves garlic, minced

- 1 teaspoon ground cinnamon

- 1/2 teaspoon ground nutmeg

- Salt and pepper to taste

Instructions:

1. Preheat the oven to 375°F (190°C).

2. Place the acorn squash halves on a baking sheet.

3. Over medium-high heat, sear the ground beef in a big skillet.

4. Cook the onion and garlic in the skillet until they are tender.

5. Stir in the cooked quinoa, cinnamon, nutmeg, salt, and pepper.

6. Spoon the beef mixture into each acorn squash half.

7. Bake for 45-50 minutes, or until the squash is tender and the filling is heated through.

Cooking Time: 60 minutes

10. Cauliflower Fried Rice

This low-carb version of fried rice uses cauliflower rice as the base, making it a great option for those following a keto or paleo diet.

Ingredients:

- 1 head cauliflower, riced

- 1 pound shrimp, peeled and deveined

- 1 red bell pepper, diced

- 1 yellow onion, diced

- 2 cloves garlic, minced

- 2 tablespoons coconut oil

- 2 tablespoons soy sauce

- 1 tablespoon sesame oil

- Salt and pepper to taste

Instructions:

1. In a large skillet, heat the coconut oil over medium-high heat.

2. Add the shrimp to the skillet and cook until pink and cooked through.

3. The shrimp should be taken out of the skillet and put aside.

4. Red bell pepper, onion, and garlic should all be added to the skillet and cooked until tender.

5. Cauliflower rice is added and heated through.

6. To the skillet, re-add the cooked shrimp.

7. Drizzle with soy sauce and sesame oil, and season with salt and pepper to taste.

8. Cook for another 2-3 minutes, stirring occasionally, until everything is heated through and well combined.

Cooking Time: 20 minutes

CHAPTER SIX

Dessert

1. Keto Chocolate Mousse

This low-carb, high-fat dessert is perfect for women over 50 who are following a ketogenic diet. It's creamy, rich, and satisfying, and can be made in just a few minutes.

Ingredients:

- 1 cup heavy cream

- 2 tbsp unsweetened cocoa powder

- 1 tsp vanilla extract

- 2 tbsp powdered erythritol

Instructions:

1. The heavy cream should be whipped until firm peaks form.

2. The whipped cream should be mixed with the chocolate powder, vanilla extract, and erythritol.

3. Mix the ingredients thoroughly by gently folding them together.

4. Place portions of the mousse in serving bowls.

5. Before serving, place in the fridge for at least 30 minutes.

Cooking time: 10 minutes

2. Coconut Chia Seed Pudding

This vegan and gluten-free dessert is perfect for women over 50 who are looking for a healthy and filling dessert option. Chia seeds are packed with fibre and healthy fats, making this pudding a nutritious and satisfying treat.

Ingredients:

- 1/4 cup chia seeds

- 1 cup coconut milk

- 1 tbsp honey

- 1 tsp vanilla extract

Instructions:

1. In a bowl, combine all the ingredients and stir thoroughly.

2. Overnight or for at least two hours, cover and chill.

3. Serve cold, topped with fresh fruit or nuts, if desired.

Cooking time: 5 minutes

3. Baked Apples with Cinnamon and Almonds

This warm and cosy dessert is perfect for a cold winter night. The combination of baked apples, cinnamon, and almonds is both comforting and delicious.

Ingredients:

*   2 apples

*   2 tbsp chopped almonds

*   1 tsp cinnamon

*   1 tbsp honey

Instructions:

1. Preheat the oven to 375°F.

2. Apples should be cored and cut in half.

3. Place the apples in a baking dish.

4. Mix the almonds, cinnamon, and honey together in a bowl.

5. Spoon the almond mixture into the apple halves.

6. Bake for 30-35 minutes, or until the apples are tender and the almond mixture is golden brown.

Cooking time: 35 minutes

4. Chocolate Avocado Pudding

This healthy and decadent dessert is perfect for women over 50 who are looking for a dairy-free and gluten-free option. The avocado adds a creamy texture, while the cocoa powder gives the pudding a rich chocolate flavour.

Ingredients:

- 2 ripe avocados

- 1/4 cup cocoa powder

- 1/4 cup honey

- 1 tsp vanilla extract

- Pinch of salt

Instructions:

1. Scoop the flesh out of the avocados and place it in a blender or food processor.

2. Add the cocoa powder, honey, vanilla extract, and salt to the blender.

3. Blend until smooth and creamy.

4. Serve chilled, topped with fresh berries or nuts, if desired.

Cooking time: 10 minutes

5. Strawberry Coconut Ice Cream

This dairy-free and sugar-free ice cream is perfect for women over 50 who are following a paleo or vegan diet.

The combination of strawberries and coconut creates a creamy and delicious dessert that's perfect for a hot summer day.

Ingredients:

- 2 cups frozen strawberries
- 1 can full-fat coconut milk
- 2 tbsp honey
- 1 tsp vanilla extract

Instructions:

1. Blend each item separately in a blender until completely smooth.

2. As directed by the manufacturer, pour the ingredients into an ice cream machine and churn.

3. Serve immediately, or freeze for later use. If frozen, let it sit at room temperature for a few minutes before scooping.

Cooking time: 10 minutes (plus time for churning in the ice cream maker)

Snack

1. Greek Yogurt with Berries and Almonds

This high-protein snack is perfect for women over 50 who are looking for a quick and easy option that will keep them satisfied until their next meal.

Ingredients:

- 1 cup plain Greek yogurt
- 1/2 cup mixed berries
- 1/4 cup sliced almonds
- 1 tsp honey (optional)

Instructions:

1. Spoon the Greek yogurt into a bowl.
2. Top with mixed berries and sliced almonds.
3. Drizzle with honey, if desired.
4. Enjoy immediately.

Cooking time: 5 minutes

2. Roasted Chickpeas

This crunchy and savoury snack is perfect for women over 50 who are looking for a healthy alternative to chips or crackers.

Ingredients:

- 1 can chickpeas, drained and rinsed

- 1 tbsp olive oil

- 1 tsp smoked paprika

- 1/2 tsp garlic powder

- Salt and pepper to taste

Instructions:

1. Preheat the oven to 400°F.

2. With a paper towel, dry the chickpeas off.

3. The chickpeas, olive oil, smoked paprika, garlic powder, salt, and pepper should all be combined in a bowl.

4. On a baking sheet, spread the chickpeas out in a single layer.

5. Bake for 20 to 25 minutes, or until golden and crispy.

6. Let cool before serving.

Cooking time: 30 minutes

3. Hard-Boiled Eggs with Avocado

This high-protein and healthy fat snack is perfect for women over 50 who are looking for a quick and satisfying option.

Ingredients:

- 2 hard-boiled eggs, peeled

- 1/2 avocado, sliced

- Salt and pepper to taste

Instructions:

1. Slice the hard-boiled eggs in half.

2. Top each half with sliced avocado.

3. Season with salt and pepper.

4. Enjoy immediately.

Cooking time: 15 minutes

4. Cottage Cheese with Pineapple and Walnuts

This high-protein and low-carb snack is perfect for women over 50 who are looking for a filling and nutritious option.

Ingredients:

- 1/2 cup cottage cheese

- 1/2 cup chopped fresh pineapple

- 1/4 cup chopped walnuts

Instructions:

1. Spoon the cottage cheese into a bowl.

2. Top with chopped pineapple and walnuts.

3. Enjoy immediately.

Cooking time: 5 minutes

5. Zucchini Chips

This healthy and low-carb snack is perfect for women over 50 who are looking for a crunchy and savoury option.

Ingredients:

- 1 large zucchini, sliced into thin rounds

- 1 tbsp olive oil

- 1 tsp garlic powder

- Salt and pepper to taste

Instructions:

1. Preheat the oven to 425°F.

2. In a bowl, mix the zucchini slices, olive oil, garlic powder, salt, and pepper together.

3. Spread the zucchini slices out in a single layer on a baking sheet.

4. Bake for ten to twelve minutes, or until crisp and golden.

5. Let cool before serving.

Cooking time: 20 minutes

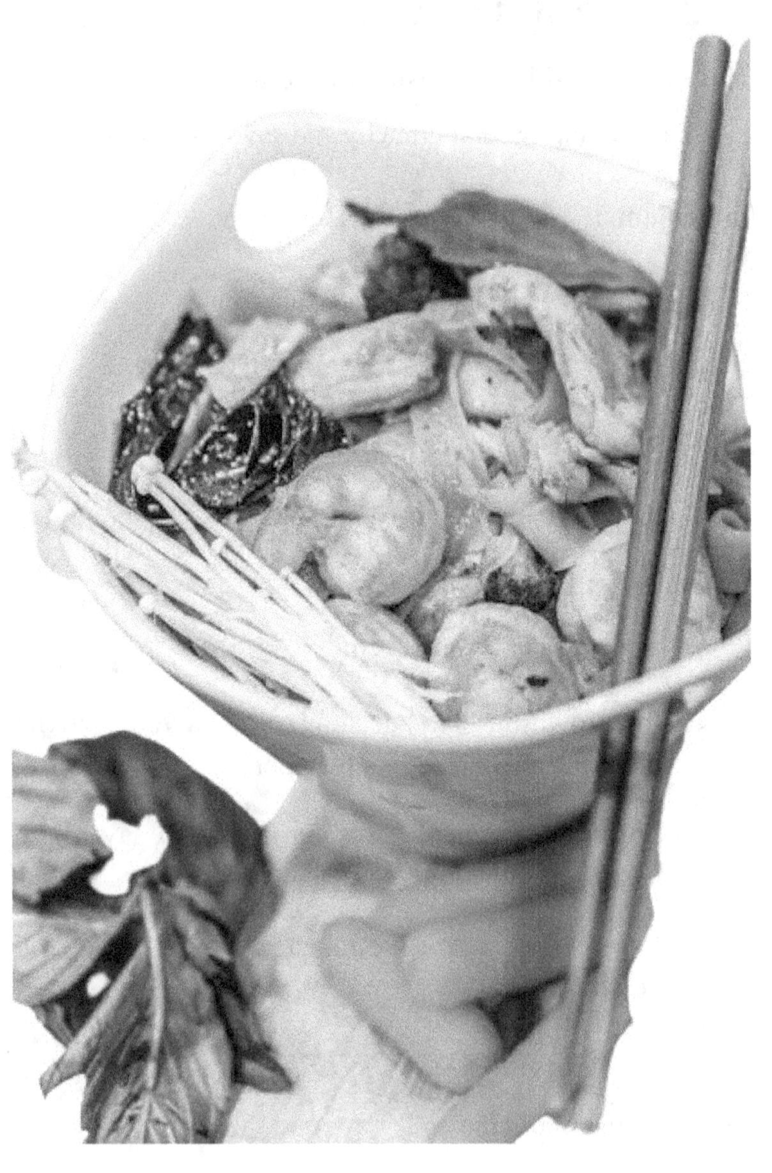

CONCLUSION

In conclusion, intermittent fasting can be an effective approach for women over 50 looking to improve their health and well-being.

This dietary strategy, which involves alternating periods of fasting and eating, has shown numerous benefits that can positively impact the lives of older women.

Firstly, intermittent fasting has been linked to weight loss and improved body composition. As women age, hormonal changes and decreased metabolic rates can make it more challenging to maintain a healthy weight.

Intermittent fasting can help overcome these obstacles by promoting fat burning and reducing overall caloric intake.

By limiting the eating window, women can naturally reduce their calorie consumption and create an energy deficit necessary for weight loss.

Furthermore, intermittent fasting has been shown to preserve lean muscle mass, which is essential for maintaining strength and mobility as women age.

Another key benefit of intermittent fasting for women over 50 is its potential to enhance metabolic health. Age-related insulin resistance and the risk of developing conditions like type 2 diabetes become more prevalent in this demographic.

Intermittent fasting has been shown to improve insulin sensitivity, regulate blood sugar levels, and lower the risk of diabetes. It also helps reduce inflammation in the body, which is associated with numerous chronic diseases.

Intermittent fasting can increase longevity and lower the incidence of age-related diseases through enhancing metabolic health.

Furthermore, intermittent fasting has been linked to cognitive benefits, which are particularly important for women over 50 who may be concerned about maintaining mental sharpness and preventing age-related cognitive decline.

Studies have shown that intermittent fasting can stimulate the production of brain-derived neurotrophic factor (BDNF), a protein that supports the growth and function of neurons.

This may enhance cognitive function, improve memory, and protect against neurodegenerative diseases such as Alzheimer's and Parkinson's.

Intermittent fasting has also been associated with improvements in cardiovascular health, another crucial aspect for women over 50.

By reducing body weight, improving insulin sensitivity, and lowering blood pressure and cholesterol levels, intermittent fasting can reduce the risk of heart disease and stroke.

These benefits can have a significant impact on overall longevity and quality of life.

While intermittent fasting offers numerous advantages for women over 50, it's essential to approach it with caution and seek guidance from healthcare professionals. Due to the physiological changes that occur with age, women may have specific nutritional needs that should be considered when implementing intermittent fasting.

Consulting with a registered dietitian or healthcare provider can ensure that nutritional requirements are met, and any potential health concerns are addressed.

In conclusion, intermittent fasting can be a valuable dietary approach for women over 50. It can help with weight management, enhance metabolic health, improve cognitive function, and promote cardiovascular well-being. However, it is crucial to approach intermittent fasting with a personalized and informed approach, taking into account individual health needs and seeking guidance from healthcare professionals.

By incorporating intermittent fasting into a balanced and healthy lifestyle, women over 50 can optimize their overall health and well-being, enabling them to enjoy a vibrant and fulfilling life.

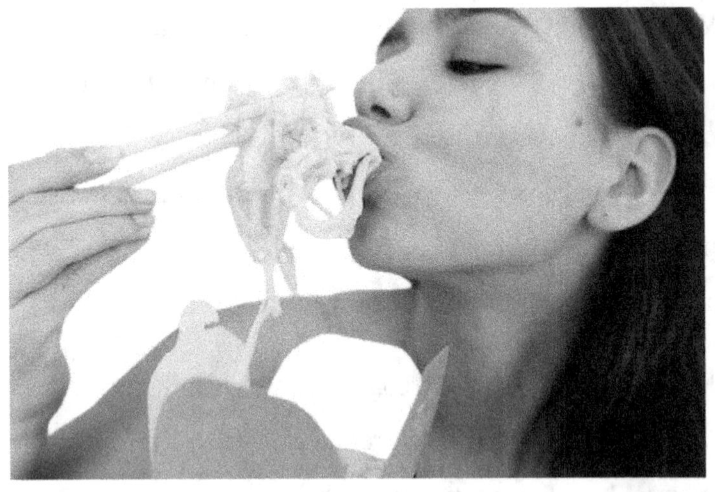

9 798885 442311